P. BALASUBRAMANIAN

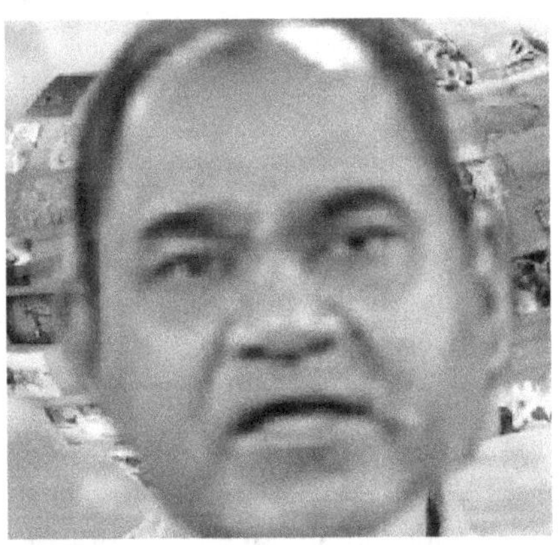

WONDER THERAPY WITH NATURE

2019

<u>*Wonder Therapy with Nature*</u>

Book Title: WONDER THERAPY WITH NATURE

Author: P.Balasubramanian

Language: English

First Edition: September 2019

Publisher: P.BALASUBRAMANIAN
                 13/5, Masilamani Colony
                 Mylapore, Chennai-600 004
                 Ph: 00914424991234/9840737555/9444175318
                 Email:
                 balasubramanian.energyaudit@gmail.com

Book size: 215 x 140 mm

No of Pages: 43

Typesetting &:   P.BALASUBRAMANIAN
Cover page

ACKNOWLEDGEMENTS

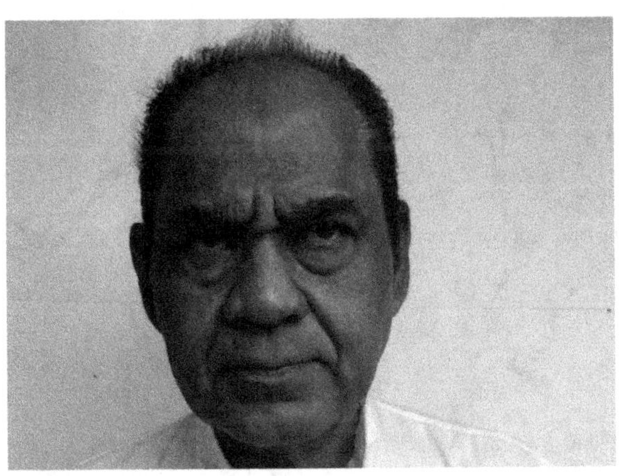

In this section, I would like to thank all the consultants and organizations for giving me generous permission to use their data in a modified form for the benefit of future generations of this world. I express our heartfelt thanks to Mr.B.Bhaskar, Editor, for the wonderful proofreading and editing.

ABOUT THE AUTHOR

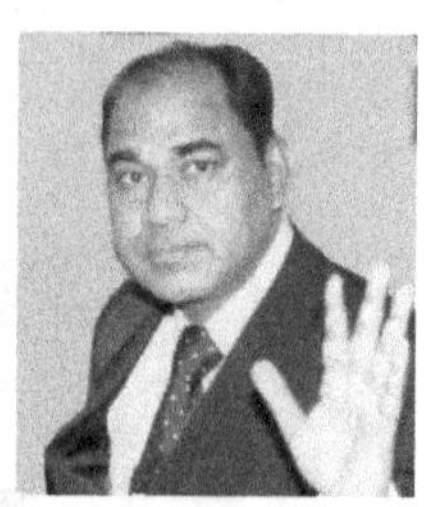

P.Balasubramanian, B.E., M.Sc.(Heat Power Engg).,
F.I.E.(India).,
LEAD AUDITOR:
ISO 50001/14001/22301/18001,
BEE Accredited Energy auditor (AEA-0105) and B.O.E
from Tamilnadu Govt.
Carries out Energy audit for industries & buildings of all
sectors.

Author of three Books on 'Energy Auditing', "Water Scarcity and Flood control "and other ten books on "Energy neuro programming" (5 in English and 5 in Tamil).

The most popular ones are 'Future with Nature', 'Success in the Digital world', 'Light the Lamp of Success', 'Cosmic Road Map of Success', 'Build a bright future with nature for your sons and daughters', 'Energy Neuro Programming (e-np)' and 'The Ultimate Gateway to Success'.

He does free counseling and support for all problems (Physical, personal, mental, emotional) using Cosmic Therapy as a service worldwide.

Holds a Doctorate in Alternate Medicine. He conducts training on personality development.

Age: 72 yrs, 50 years experience in SPIC, BHEL, Saudi ARAMCO, SEPL. 25 years in service to humanity
Address: 13/5, Masilamani Colony, Mylapore, Chennai-600004, India
Telefax: 0091-44-2499 1234, Mobile: 09444175318 / 09840737555

Email: balasubramanian.energyaudit@gmail.com
Website: www.poweraudit.co
Blog: www.digitalenergysuccess.blogspot.com

FOREWORD

I have written this book with the intention that people of the world should get the benefit of this wonderful gift of God everyone has already got in their hands but do not know it. With little resources at my command, I have written this book. My intention is to serve the people of the whole world who have helped me a lot when I was there in their country for work. I could not resist the temptation of sharing this tested knowledge with all my brothers and sisters in the world. This technique is a simple and practical one, and can be learnt in a minute. The secret is to keep one's hands on the affected parts until the problem is solved. I have explained all the common diseases faced by mankind including the sexual problems as a ready reckoner. This is a universal method, which can be followed by anyone from the age of 20 to 100 years. There is no nationality, religion, caste, creed, gender and language involved in this system. I teach this new technique after trying it on thousands of people throughout the world. At the age of 72 years, I am hale and healthy only because of cosmic energy therapy. This system only complements allopathy medicines patients take. Success will come if the cosmic therapy is integrated with their lifestyle. Do not underestimate it just because it seems simple. It is a scientific system. Do not do cosmic therapy for others out of anxiety. Ask them to do it by themselves by educating them. First of all, you have to increase your own energy level to a higher level, so that you have more immunity to diseases and develop resistance power. Practice is the secret. If any assistance is required, please send an email or phone me. I shall be happy to help you after scanning you over the phone. I shall send you my e-books on cosmic therapy free of cost to enrich your knowledge, which could give you more confidence and satisfaction. Do not get over enthusiastic and then advise people to stop the treatment they are undertaking.

P.BALASUBRAMANIAN

TABLE OF CONTENTS

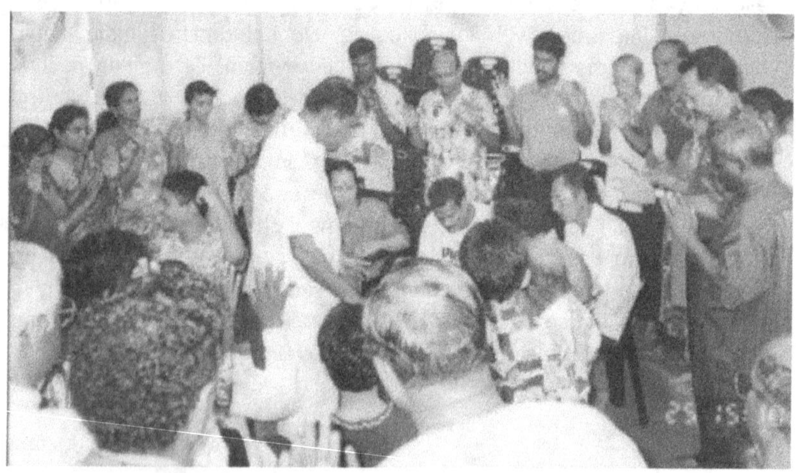

1. INTRODUCTION

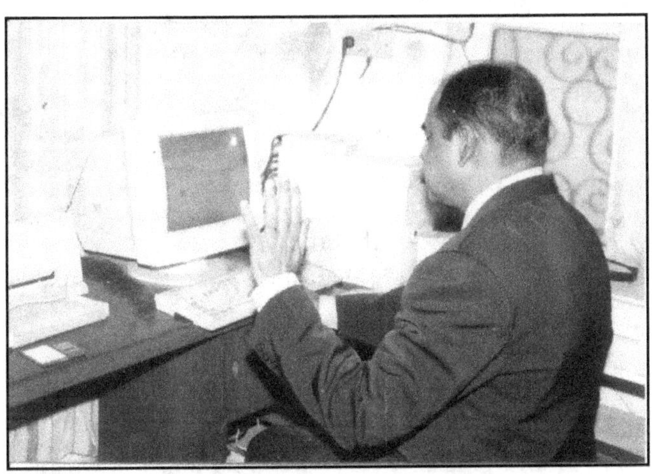

We live in a digital era. There are multiple problems facing mankind today, which were non-existent before. Moreover, as we move towards higher technology, we need higher touch to withstand the stresses of the modern world.

Why don't people change?

This question had always rung in my ears. Why don't people change even after reading many self-development books and undergoing many management-training programmes?

They may seriously try it for a maximum of one week and then discontinue it.

My formula:

Hence, my formula is: Energy + Thought = Success.

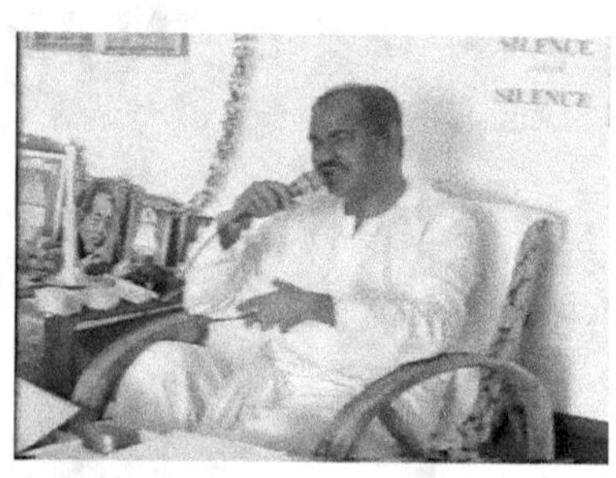

Keep your hands on affected parts with intention. You will achieve success.

The advantages of this method are:-

1. One can do it anywhere, viz. while talking, watching TV and even while travelling.

2. No rituals and   methodologies are involved

3. It is a scientific system

4. This gift is in everybody's hands. For all problems, just keep the hands on the body.

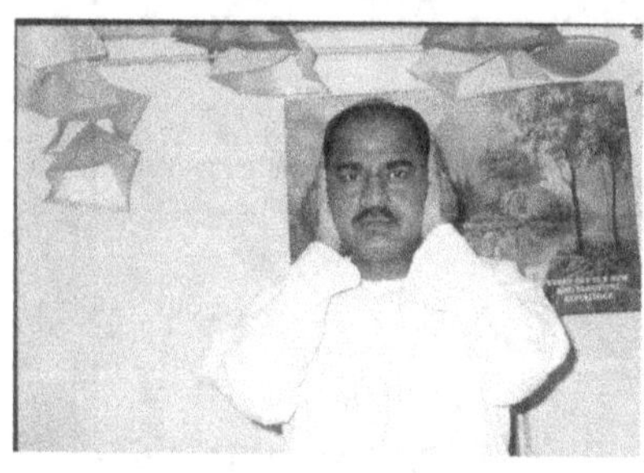

It had transformed many others and me. Hence, I give here the benefit of this experience to all the citizens of this world.

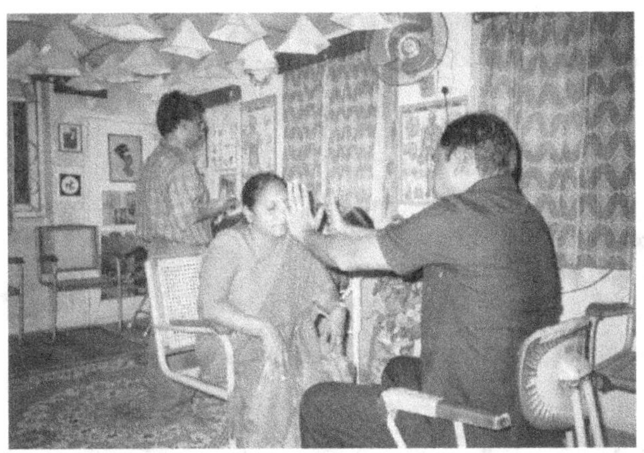

How to Succeed Using this Book

Follow the three steps below.

1. Follow the lifestyle tips, e.g.

    a. Chew food & eat slowly

    b. Physical activity

    c. Diet control

3. Cosmic Therapy

    a. Pass cosmic energy to your body system.

    Mind then becomes calm and works smarter.

Jobs become simpler and easier if the steps given in this book are followed. You can slowly improve upon your skills and fine-tune your body and mind. Be assured that by following the tips, you can truly improve your working in all fronts.

A Quick Glance through the Whole Book

1. Do cosmic therapy in the appropriate places (head, front, back, top, heart, stomach, end of spinal cord). Wherever there is physical problem, simply touch the appropriate places with intention.

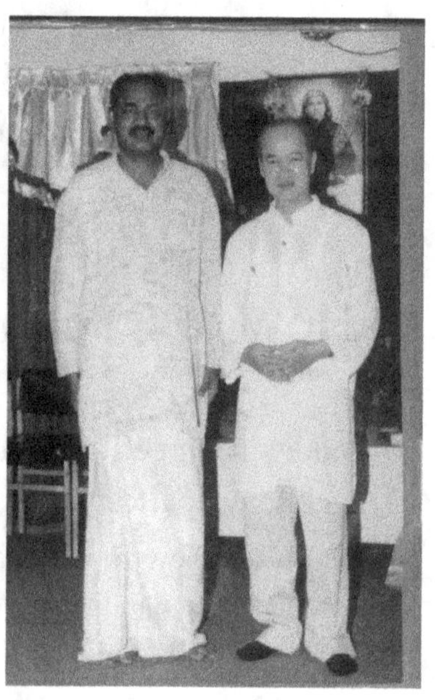

2. Do physical activities daily (exercises, walking or doing household chores).

* Chew the food slowly and eat slowly.

* Eat the right food

3. A sound mind in a sound body

When this is achieved, your mind will automatically search for the appropriate knowledge.

2. This is the Digital World

Do You Yearn for Success?

Practising cosmic therapy daily gives stress-free life and you will be able to cope better with the fast paced world. Your skills will be sharpened and you will be able to achieve your goals of life.

Go through sections viz. Life audit, courses in my website for more information.

www.poweraudit.co

www.digitalenergysuccess.blogspot.com

If cosmic energy is practised regularly, you can get healthy body, mind and spirit. Cosmic energy dissolves everything that creates tension, unpleasantness and fatigue. You can achieve your goals and ambitions using cosmic energy. Cosmic energy helps to increase energy and creative power.

See videos and other photos by clicking the links below.

http://www.poweraudit.co/videos.html

www.digitalenergysuccess.blogspot.com

3. Problems faced by all

If this chapter alone is followed, success is yours in no time. See the images and keep your hands at the appropriate places as per your problems. Practice is the secret. Keep your hands until the problem is solved. You can do it while travelling, watching TV or lying down. As you practice cosmic therapy, you will start to appreciate it better. The common problems faced by men and women are: -

1. Lack of concentration
2. Injuries
3. Fear
4. Memory Power
5. Injury
6. Lack of self-confidence/Success
7. Eye pain
8. Low Energy and tiredness
9. Stress and sleep
10. Digestion
11. Concentration
12. Depresssion
13. Pain

Hand positions for some of the diseases are shown below for quick reference, and if this alone is followed, success will come quickly.

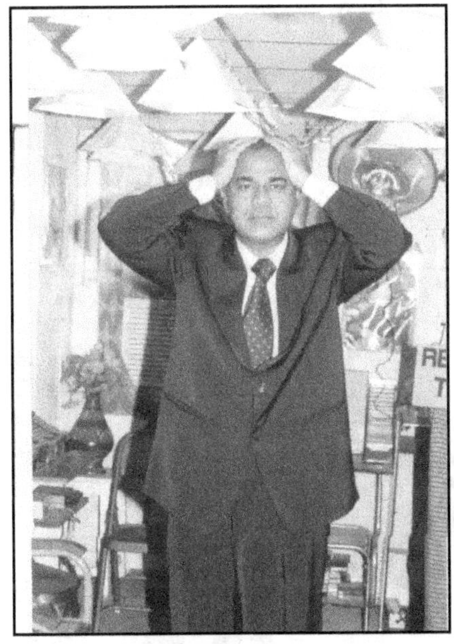

Memory Power, Hairfall

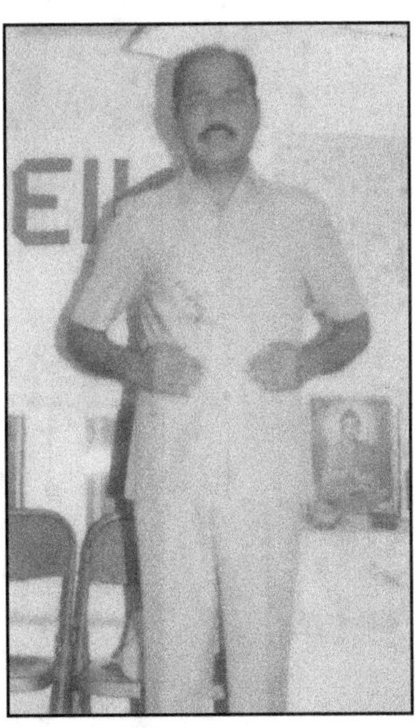

Digestion

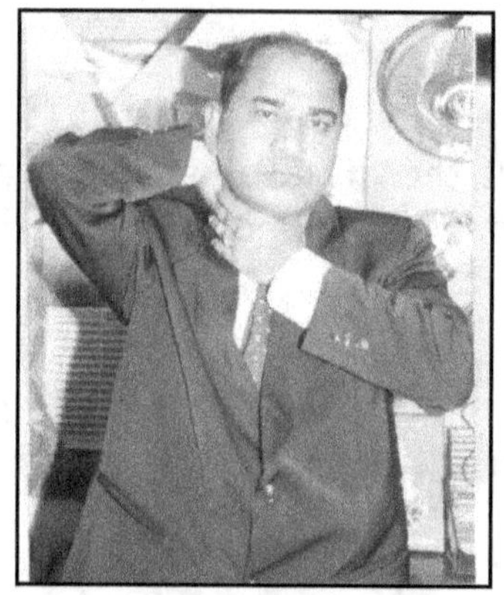

**Lack of self-confidence,
Success**

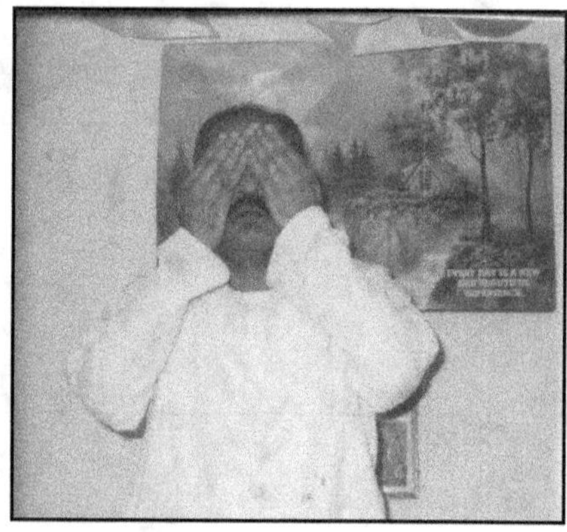

Eye pain

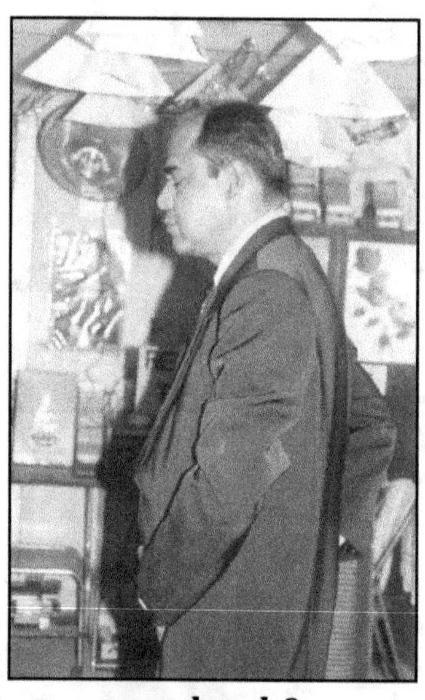

**Low energy level &
Tireness**

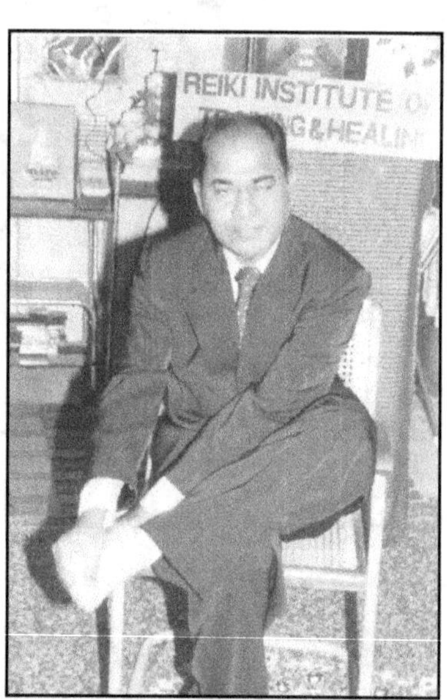

Injury

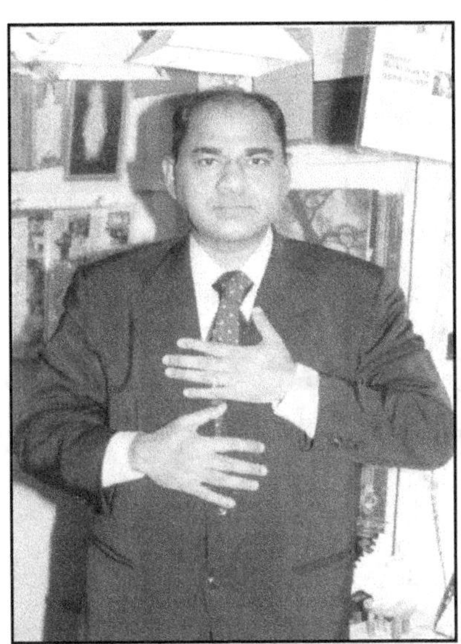

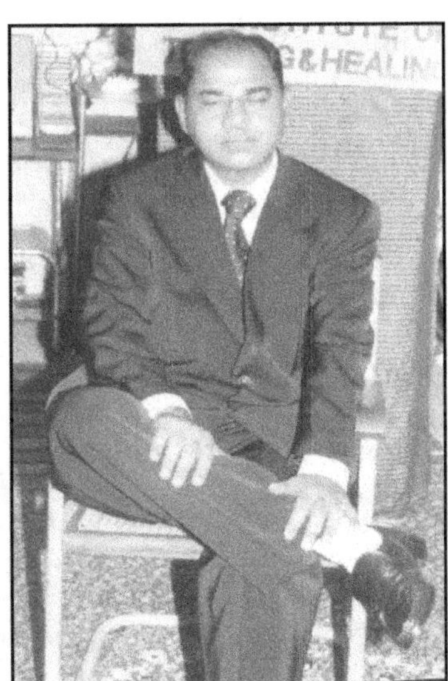

Exam fear, insomnia and stress   **Pain in legs**

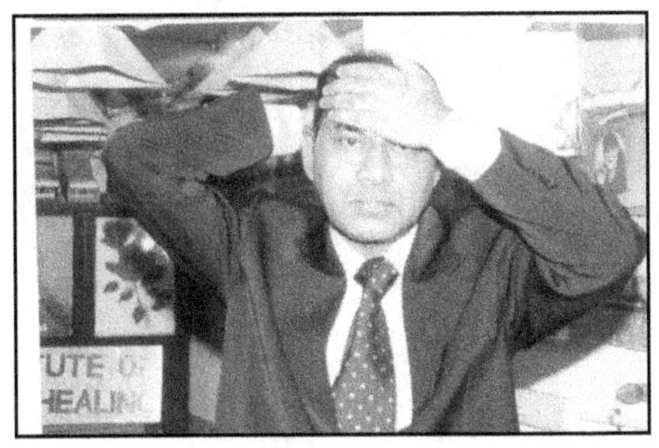

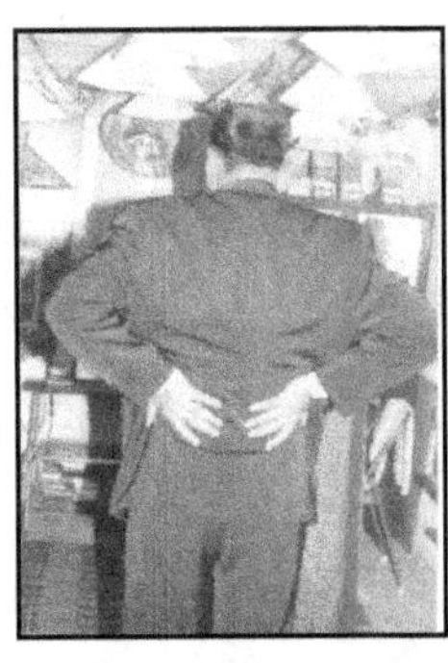

**Keep hands on forehead and back head.
As you practice, your concentration
power will improve**

Pain in the back

I will give solutions one by one to all the problems facing the present generation.

1. Memory Power

This is a common problem for all.

Solution: Keep the hand on the right and left side of the brain as shown in the photo.

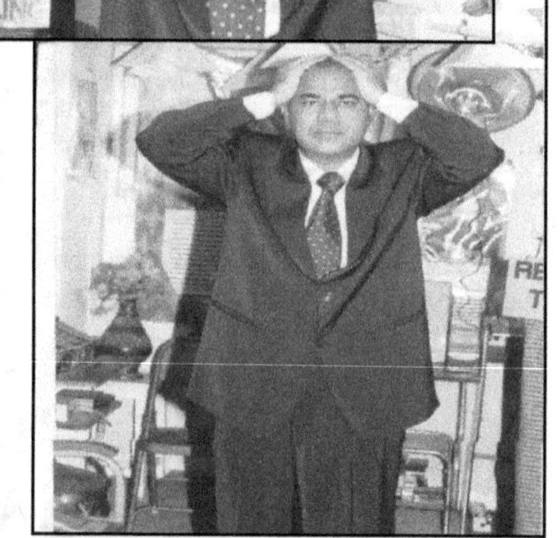

2. Lack of Concentration

This is a common problem faced by all.

Students are not able to concentrate, as there are many distractions. When they are studying, many thoughts come and interfere. For concentration power, we have to activate the pituitary gland further. The pituitary gland is in the forehead. Keep the hand on the forehead and on the back head. When the forehead is activated, the pituitary gland gets charged. The pituitary gland, which is called the master gland, secretes ten different types of hormones. The face becomes bright, clarity of thinking improves and one is able to concentrate better. Everything comes only by practice. Hence, practise, practise, and practise!

Solution: Keep your hands on forehead and back head as shown in the photo

3. Injuries

Everyone commonly encounter sprains, stiff muscles and bruises. They can heal these on their own. For example, if a person has got sprain in the left knee, he can keep his hands on the knee with intention. When you keep the hand on the knee, the energy goes there and removes the blockages. They have to keep the hand until the pain goes. Suppose you have stiffness in your calf muscles, you only have to keep your hand on the calf muscles. The heat of the hand automatically removes muscular tension. The same thing applies to bruises as well.

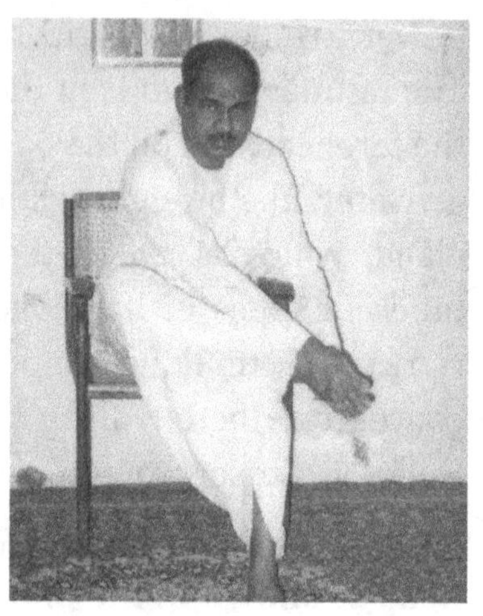

Solution: Keep your hands on the affected parts until the pain goes.

4. Fear, Stress and sleep

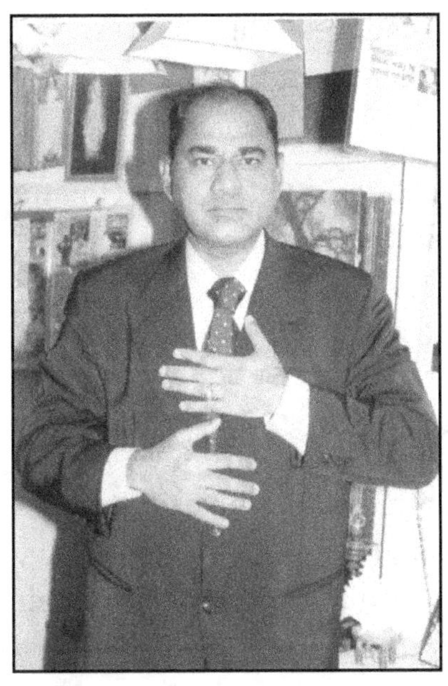

Stress and tension are common to all. In all these problems, the common denominator is to keep one's hands on the affected part. The stresses are of two types; one is emotional stress, another is mental stress. For emotional stress, one has to keep one hand on the heart and the other hand on the stomach, just above the navel. The energy goes to the heart and stomach, which are the emotional centres of the body. When the energy reaches it, the fear goes. Cosmic energy has released the blockage. Regarding mental stress, 'mental' signifies the brain. The person has to keep his hand on his head and pass energy until the tension is released. When you keep the hand on the affected part, the warmth in the hand opens the blood vessels and improves blood circulation. The secretion of the lactate comes down. The more the secretion of lactate, the more the tension level. So when one keeps the hand there, the tension comes down. When the tension level comes down, you will feel calm, as your head becomes light.

Some people do not get good sleep due to stress. For this, they have to keep their hands on the heart and the stomach.

Solution: Keep the hands on the heart and stomach as shown in the photo.

5. To improve Self-confidence

Many people do not have faith in themselves. They feel they are inferior. This may be due to past trauma they may had experienced. This trauma remains in their subconscious mind. Passing the cosmic energy to the head can remove this. If they practise for three days, the past trauma will easily disappear and they will feel confident.

Solution: Keep the hands on the right and left side of head.

6.Eye pain

Many wear glasses. Eyestrain and headache are inter-related. For eye pain, energise the eyes by passing cosmic energy to the eyes. This is called palming technique. When you gently keep your hands

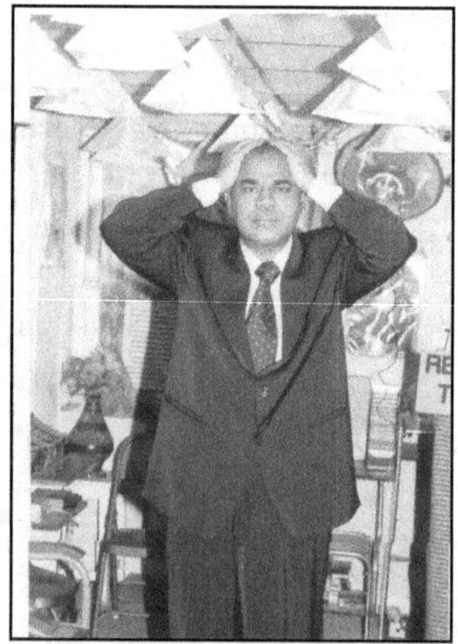

on your eyes, cosmic energy goes to the eyes and the strain reduces.

Besides this, you can practise neck and eye exercises. The neck and eye muscles are inter-connected. The eye and neck movement exercises involve up and down, sideways movement and rotation (clockwise and anti-clockwise) of the eyes and neck. Then, facial massage can also be done. Gentle stroking can be done on the eyebrows. If the headache is on the top of the head, keep your hand on the head.

Solution: Palming of the eyes with both hands as shown in thephoto.

7. For professional success

Solution: Keep the hands on the front throat and the back throat.

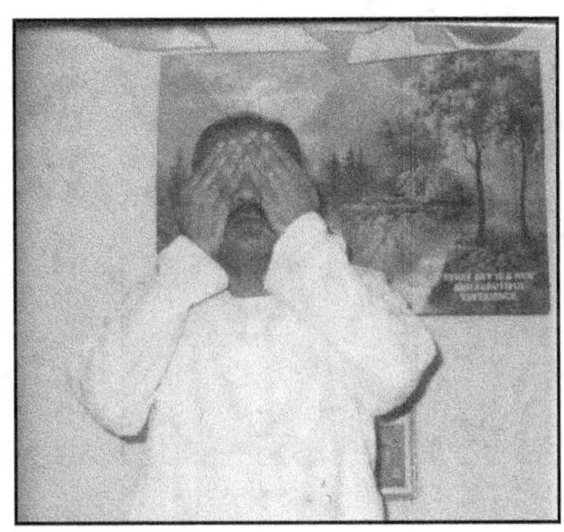

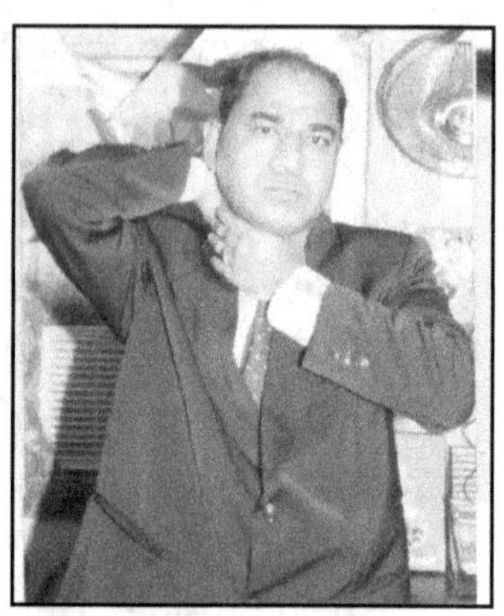

8. Indigestion

Indigestion is a common problem for all. You should keep both your hands on both sides of the stomach.

Avoid junk food and spicy food. Chew the food and eat. Do not eat anything when you are not hungry.

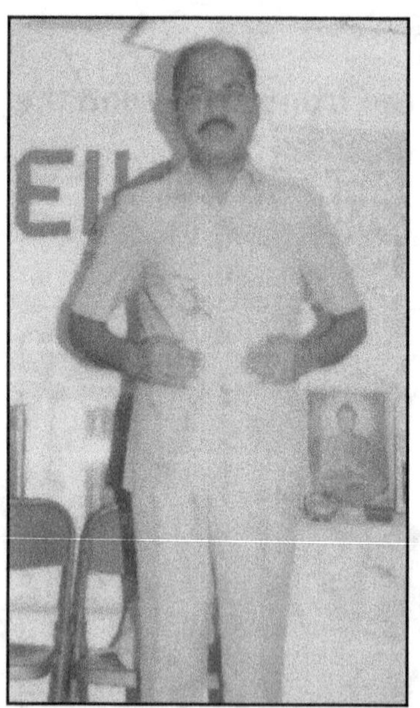

9. Depression

The other stress-related problem is depression. People refer to depression as

22

spirit work or evil forces. In fact, there is no such thing as spirits or evil forces. The blocked-up emotions are the cause of the problems. When we apply positive cosmic energy, it removes the negative energy. Some people call this negative energy or evil forces. Cosmic therapy has removed depression for quite a number of

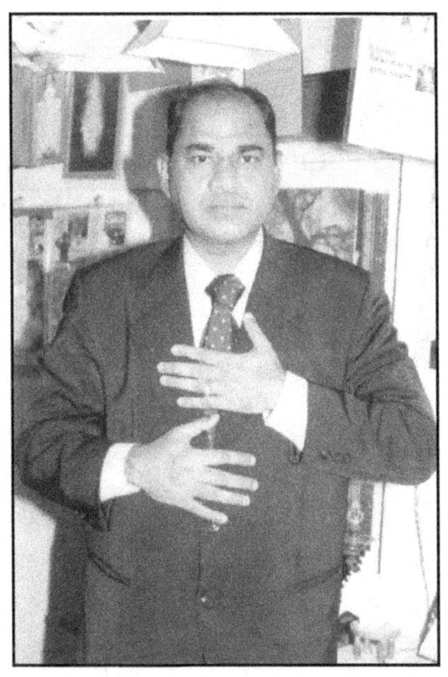

people. One out of four people, who come to see me, suffer from this type of disease. All age groups of people, right from children of five years upto eighty years, suffer from psychosomatic diseases.

With cosmic therapy, a person can heal himself. It has helped so many people. The moment depression is released the physical problem vanishes. People who come to me with back pain and neck pain feel better when depression is released. Depression is the source of many diseases. Even some skin diseases come from emotional problems.

Solution: Keep your hands on heart and stomach until you are calm and quiet.

10. Tiredness

Keep your hands on the urinary bladder and the end of spinal cord.

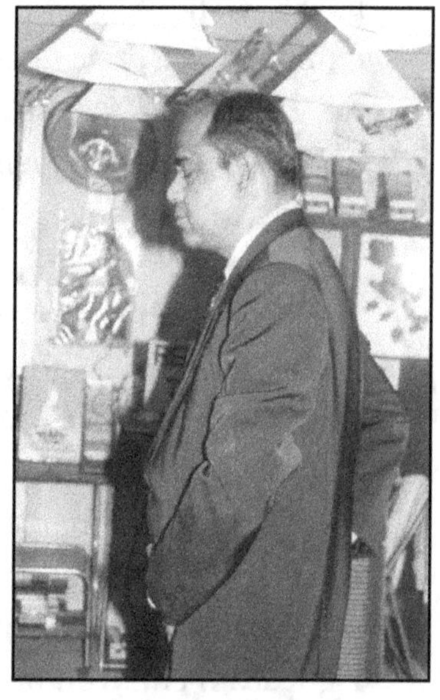

11.Asthma

Bronchial Asthma: Occurs when the bronchial vessels are blocked.
Cardiac Asthma: Occurs when the chest is affected by attacks.

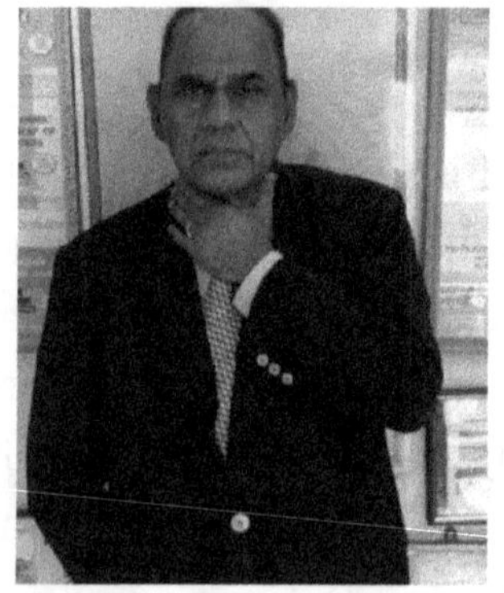

Renal

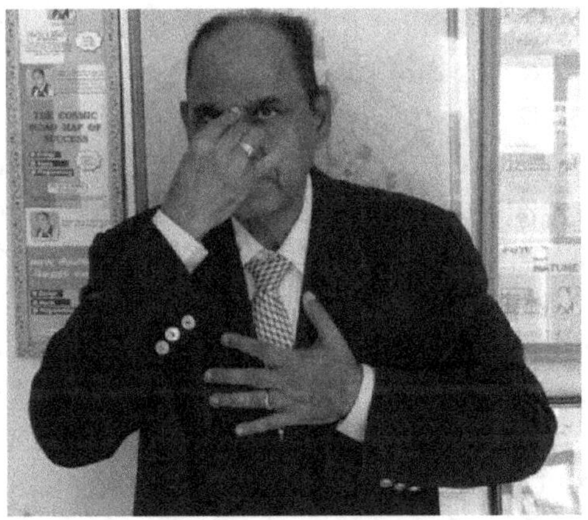

Asthma: Problem in kidneys and its consequent affliction.

Asthma, in general, is the shrinking of the respiratory organs that result in decreased supply of air to the liver, which result in palpitation and suffocation.

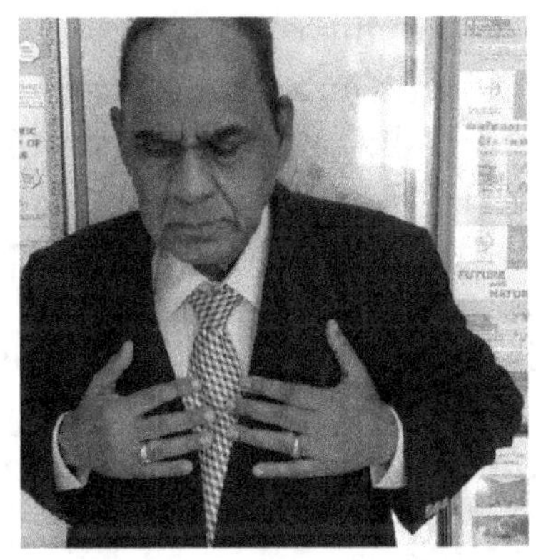

Reasons for Asthmatic Attacks

1. Dust and living in unhygienic conditions;
2. Improper food habits;
3. Drinking of liquor and smoking habits;
4. Intake of meat everyday;

5. Excessive consumption of cold drinks, ice cream and taking stale food.

In other cases, like constant exposure to dust and smoke, it becomes imperative to advise the person to avoid that constant exposure, apart from cosmic energy therapy. Some may be allergic to cold water. To cure these people, infusing cosmic energy into them can strengthen the thyroid and the para-thyroid glands. This removes the blocks in these parts and the relieved person can take cold water from then on. Though placing hands on the thyroid and para thyroid glands along with the hands on the chest effectively curtails **asthma, placing one hand on the front throat and the other on the chest ensures a quick recovery.**

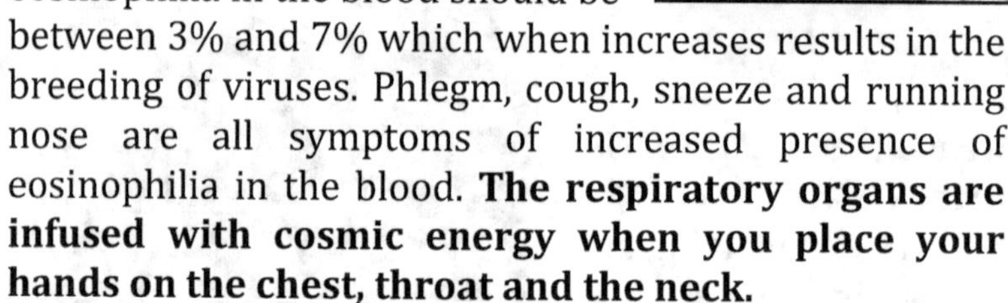

12. Eosinophilia

On an average, the presence of eosinophilia in the blood should be between 3% and 7% which when increases results in the breeding of viruses. Phlegm, cough, sneeze and running nose are all symptoms of increased presence of eosinophilia in the blood. **The respiratory organs are infused with cosmic energy when you place your hands on the chest, throat and the neck.**

13. Diabetes

The carbohydrate content in the food we eat gets digested and mixes with the blood in the form of glucose.

The normal level of glucose in a sample of 100ml of blood is 80 to 120 mgm, but this increases to 120-160 mgm when we take food. When the normal limit is exceeded, the excess glucose is excreted with urine. To contain this increased level of glucose in the blood, the gland secretes insulin through its beta cells. This insulin clears the excessive glucose present and coats the walls of the liver as glycogen, which induces strength to the cells. Diabetes occurs when the beta cells of the gland get affected in some way, thus preventing it from secreting the required insulin in the blood.

Two Kinds of Diabetes

1. Diabetes caused by lack of insulin – which can be corrected by injecting insulin into the blood.
2. Diabetes caused by factors other than insulin, which can be controlled by diet and medicines.

Symptoms

Diabetes has chance to strike when the person feels the following symptoms: frequent urination, dizziness, giddiness, fatigue, frequent hunger and thirst, loss of weight, itching sensation in the body, irritation in the reproductive organs, tired legs or an injury not healed for quite a long time. When any of the symptoms occurs, it is advisable to test the blood for sugar. In confirmed cases, proper medicines along with **cosmic energy therapy (placing one hand on the chest and the other on the belly) can be adopted to control it.**

14.Impotency

I have come across many a childless couple that has successfully tasted everything else in life. Though population explosion is the much-hyped issue worldwide, many still suffer from the issue of childlessness.

Many couples come forward to learn cosmic energy therapy to cure them and bear a child. A man's sperm should be productive and capable of passing the live cells into a woman's womb. Similarly, the woman's ovum should be a full-grown egg and the tube to the womb free of blocks. Further, the womb should be strong and devoid of any other problems.

Cosmic energy therapy demands treatment to the adrenal (kidneys), pituitary (forehead) organs and the end of spinal cord.

Kegel exercises are a simple exercise to strengthen sexual organs. This will strengthen your pelvic floor, vaginal muscles and organs.
To do this, stop urinating midstream. The muscles you use to do this are your pelvic floor muscles. Your testicles will also rise when you contract these muscles.
Now that you know where these muscles are, contract them for 5 to 20 seconds. Then release them.
Repeat this exercise 10 to 20 times in a row, three to four times a day.

Exercise for the Anus Muscles

Contracting and releasing of anus muscles daily 30 times a day in the morning, evening and night will strengthen the urinary bladder, pelvic and vaginal muscles and organs. Feel that air is entering via anus.

Cosmic touch for organs

Men: Do cosmic therapy for penis, testicles, and urinary bladder by holding them for 10 minutes for three times a day

Women: Do cosmic therapy for Vagina, Uterus by touching them for 10 minutes for three times a day.

This has worked for many people when medicines fail to arrest urination.

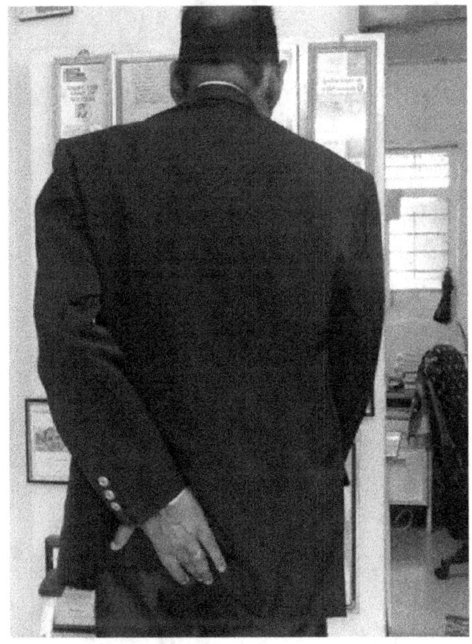

15.Headache

Millions of people around the world suffer from headache, which leaves them bedridden. Headache, generally, falls under two categories,

(1) Primary, that includes migraine

(2) Secondary that befalls on lack of metabolism and the presence of toxins in the blood.

If you keep your hands on your head and stomach, your headache will disappear.

16.Menopause

Menopause is nothing but a biological change that occurs in women due to the reduced secretion of estrogen and progesterone glands. Normally occurring during 40 to 50 years of age, this menopause and the consequent pain can be effectively curtailed by **cosmic energy therapy by keeping the hands on the uterus and organs.**

17. For Pregnant Women

Pregnant women, when subjected to cosmic energy therapy, can feel vividly the baby's movement in their womb. Even unborn and newborn babies can be cosmically energised. The most important impact is that these cosmically energised pregnant women are not prone to mental depression at any point of time. A psychological boost in confidence and courage is necessary for healthy delivery of the baby, and cosmic energy ensures just this conducive environment on pregnant women.

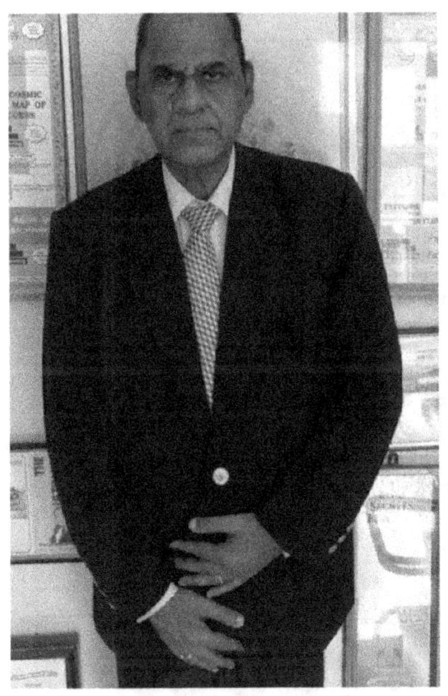

Premenstrual syndrome, the last stage before menses, results in excessive irritation and fatigue.

If problems occur on these parts, **placing hands on the uterus and the organ will solve the problem.**

18. Women's Menses problems

Cosmic energy

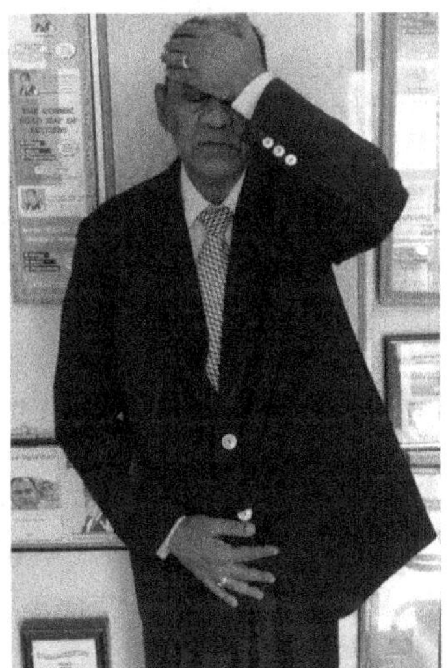

therapy should be more intensely practised during the menses, as extra effort is needed to complement the body when it sheds its
impurities. The menses may not be normal for many women with some complaining of excessive discharge of blood and pain. But cosmic energy, being a natural therapy in itself, effectively controls this problem. The parts where **hands can be placed to treat include the womb, reproductive organs, end of spinal cord and forehead.**

19.Heart

The muscles of the heart weigh less than half-a-kilo and it is this small piece of muscle that beats 70 times per minute when we are at rest. It distributes 5 litres of blood through the long blood vessels to the entire body enriching fifty million tissues along the way.

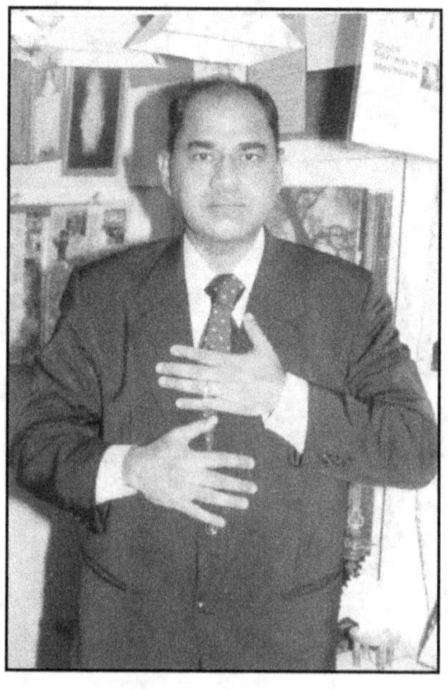

Heart pain is caused when cosmic energy is not properly channelised into the heart's energy centre. This can be effectively curtailed when cosmic energy is channelised to the heart's energy centres.

The reasons for such kind of heart ailments include tense situations, friction between relatives or emotional involvement in such situations. These factors block the heart's energy centres and hinder the flow of cosmic energy. Even when the blood flow is smooth, insufficient supply of cosmic energy creates blocks in the heart's muscles, blood vessels and valves. Channelise cosmic energy to these affected parts and you will feel the positive difference with smooth flow of blood and energy, and thus, enjoy a fresh lease of energy and life.

Place one of your hands either on the heart (situated on the left side of your chest) or its energy

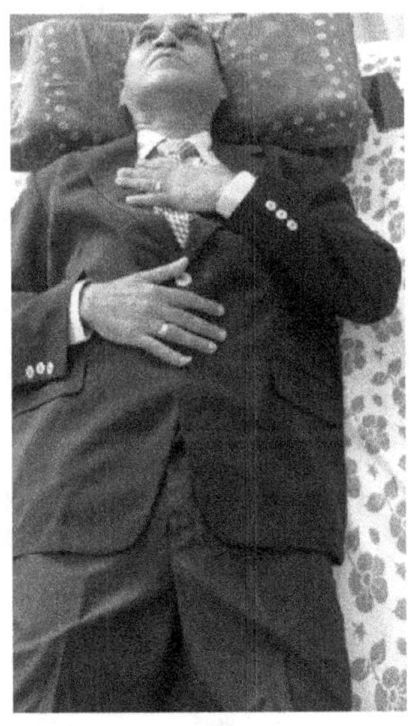

centre and the other hand on the stomach. The period for which this treatment should be continued varies according to the intensity of the ailment and pain. Hence, this treatment may be continued till one finds a comfortable and positive change and relief from pain.

It can be done as many times as possible. This placing of hands can be adopted irrespective of posture, whether sitting, lying down or even during telephonic conversation. It is a natural and universal therapy sans injections, pills, medicines, tonics, pain, side effects or the important cost factor. You merely pass the cosmic energy through your hand to the afflicted parts. That's about it!

Though yoga and meditation are as good as this therapy in treating these ailments, the lack of time and effort in adopting strict yoga postures and meditation techniques prevent us from benefiting fully. But this therapy does not demand an exclusive timetable and can effectively be inserted into one's course of actions and day-to-day activities.

20.Osteoporosis

Osteoporosis reduces the density of the bones, pushing them to become fragile and easily breakable. Hence old people, especially women, are prone to excessive damage in the hipbones, leg or hand and get fractures when they lose balance and fall. These accidents leave old people completely bedridden, throwing their lives out of gear. The bones gain weight only between 20 and 30 years of age. After this period, as the age increases, 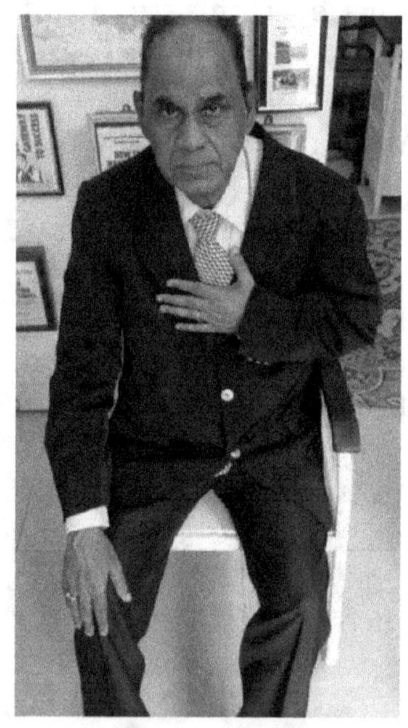 the bones are exposed to the wear and tear stage of life. Women, particularly after menopause, are severely exposed to this stage and their bones lose considerable weight.

Lack of Calcium and Vitamin D in the food intake further aggravates the situation and may lead to immediate and high degree of fractures when accidents occur. Women are comparatively exposed nearly 8% more to this osteoporosis than men are. By increasing the Estrogen level and taking calcium-rich foods such as milk, vegetables and fish, women can get resistance power by their bones getting strengthened. Speaking cosmically, **placing one's hands on the end of spinal cord infuses cosmic energy to treat osteoporosis.**

21.Arthritis

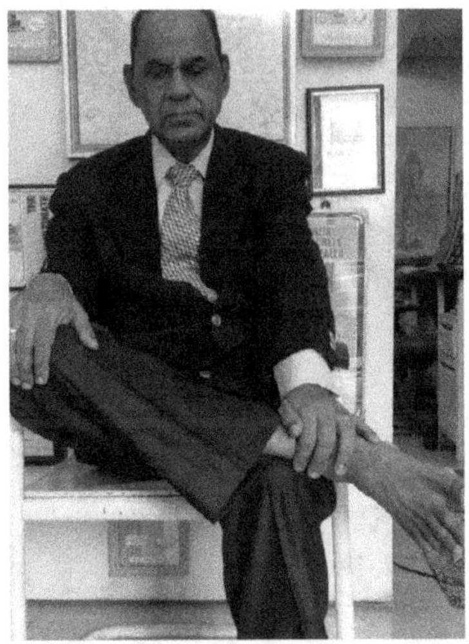

According to the World Health Organisation, nearly 360 million of people are affected by arthritis around the globe. Physically, a tissue called the cartilage, which secretes the synovial hormones on its outer walls, covers two ends of a bone. The joints present in the body of a person include the finger joints, wrist, ankle, shoulders, thighs, knees, the feet, thumbs, the joints on the neck and hip joints. Affliction of these joints is termed arthritis.

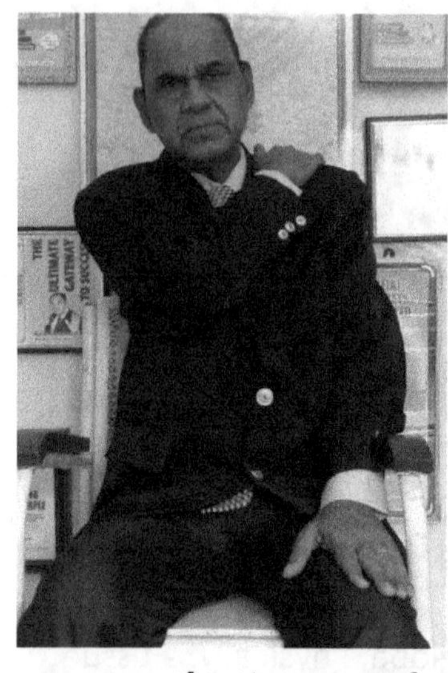

Rheumatoid Arthritis

Termed as inflammation of the joints, this autoimmune disease in arthritis occurs due to lack of resistance in the body. The rogue antibodies produced by the immune system consume the tissues and erode them. This is called a richman's disease. **By keeping hands on the heart and kidneys, the problem can be managed.**

22.Hairfall

Hairfall is one of the most common problems one faces today. Women in particular attach great importance to hair and little standing

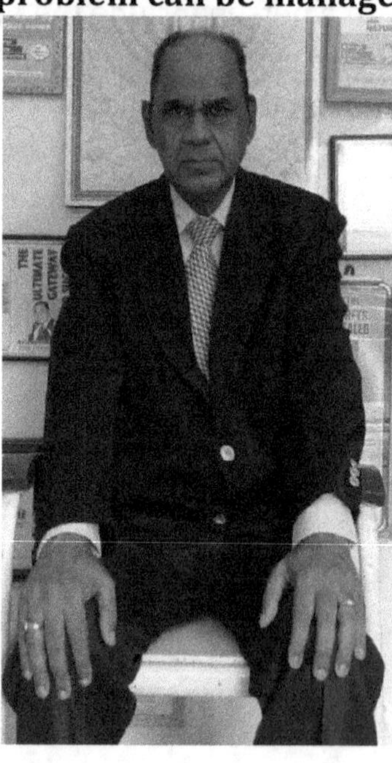

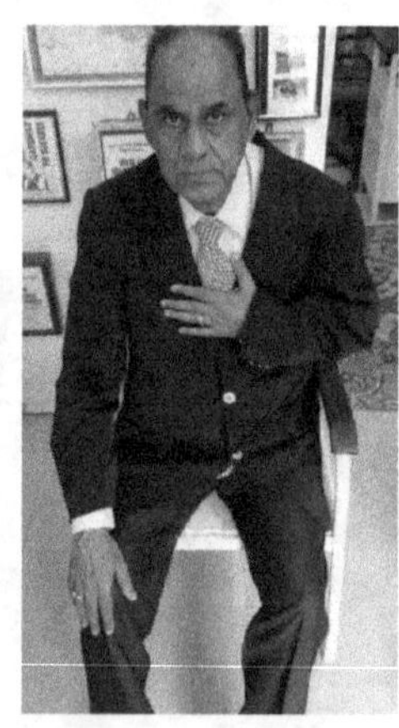

spend their available time before mirrors

and lamenting on the loss of hair. The source of hairfall again goes to mental depression, lack of iron and vitamins. When **cosmic energy is channelised on the head by placing hands on it**, the blood flow increases and once more rekindles growth of the hair. But practice holds the key to positive results. Baldness, partial hair loss and improper hair growth are common afflictions.

23. Eye Problems

The eye is a vital organ in the human body. Normally, a person blinks 22 times a minute, but when he watches TV or works at the computer, this blinking rate is considerably reduced, resulting in eye problems. The more time you spend before a TV or a computer screen, the more your blinking rate gets reduced, creating a sensation of heat on the eyes. This results in the drying up of eyes, squint eyes and pain. Reading in a lying position may also cause eye problems.

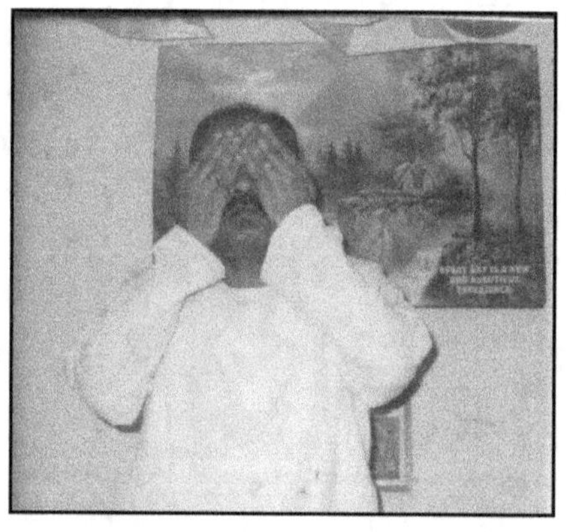

Contrary to the popular misconception that cosmic energy should not be infused into the eye; **cosmic energy can be channelised in the eyes too. This does no harm. In fact, cosmic energy cures glaucoma, the one-eye vision of Lazy eye and other eye problems.** A continuous practice of cosmic energy therapy strengthens the eyes, and spectacles can be avoided. Even cataracts in the eyes are cured by this therapy and it further lessens the impact of the eye diseases as well. Hence infusion of cosmic energy cures all eye-related problems.

24. Insomnia

Insomnia leaves a man sleepless for days together. A rich man is more exposed to this condition as he is ever filled with umpteen problems and evasive solutions. Many people, irrespective of their status, consume liquor and other intoxicants to attract sleep, but the only effect is the deterioration of health.

Placing one hand on the heart's energy centre and the other on the stomach gives the yearning soul good sleep. The reason for placing a hand on the heart's energy centre is that it is the abode of countless problems, tensions and depression. And the stomach is the centre of anger and its subsequent causes and miseries. When the hand is placed on these areas, negative factors decrease and perish, and is replaced by sleep-inducing positive factors. The mind is tranquillised and made to rest and sleep. **Placing both the hands on the chest and stomach creates an ambiance of equilibrium in one's emotions.** The most comfortable aspect of this therapy is it can be done even in a lying position. When negative vibrations come down, sleep embraces a man, and peace is born.

25.Skin

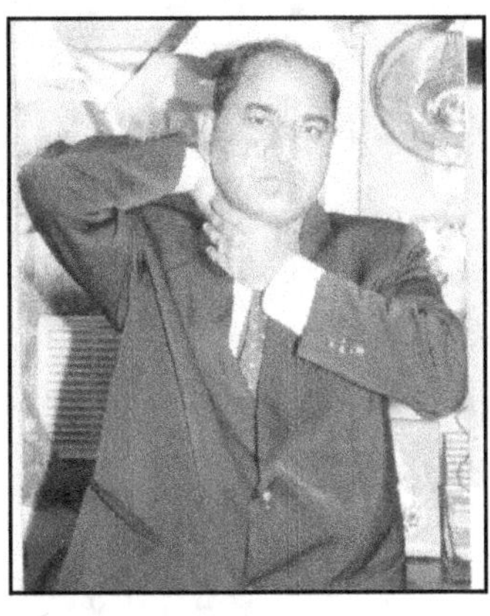

The longest part of the body, the skin, is 175 sq.m in breadth and ½ cm thick. The blood vessels and nerves are cojoined together and control the heat of the body. The sweat acts as an exit to keep the body heat in equilibrium. Skin diseases like rashes, dry skin, pimples, cracks, contraction, lack of nutrition, freshness, irritation and other irregularities can be dealt with by **placing of hands on the throat and kidneys to infuse cosmic energy.**

26.Sinusitis

This occurs by the formation of fluids in the sinus area of the nose. Irregularity in the inner tissues and flesh may also lead to sinusitis. **Cosmic energy therapy requires the placing of fingers on either side of the nose's bones and infusing cosmic energy into it, followed by placing of hands on the front and rear portions of the throat and neck.**

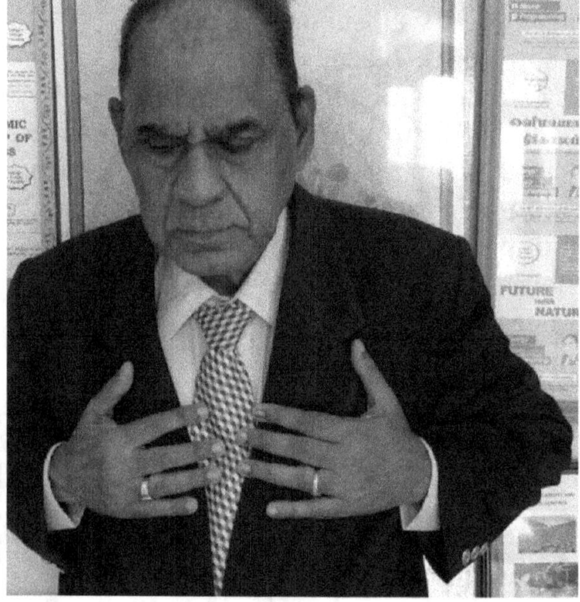

27. Tooth pain

For pain in teeth and gums, just keep the fingertips on the face where there is pain in the

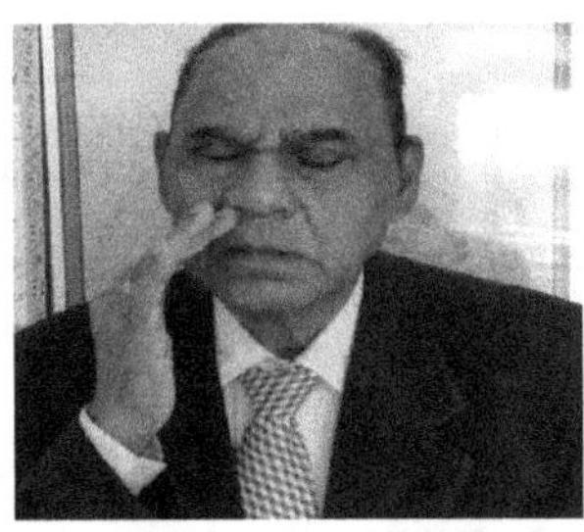

teeth. It will go away just like that. I did not know this before. When I kept my finger on the face, the pain went off within 2 minutes. Had I known this before, I would not have removed the wisdom teeth on one side. Now I am managing with wisdom teeth only on one side. Cosmic therapy is a really great method!

28.Pain in the ears

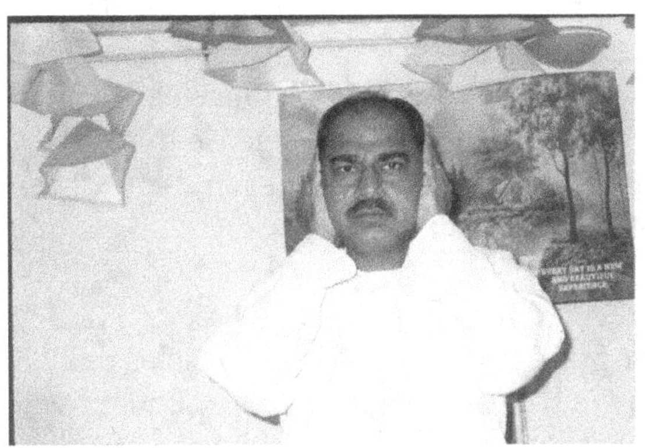

For pain the ears and inside, keep the palm over the ears . Pain will go.

29.Frequent urination (urinary incontinence)

This is a common problem for many people.

Kegel exercises are a simple exercise to stop frequent urination. This will strengthen your pelvic floor muscles. To do this, stop urinating midstream. The muscles you use to do this are your pelvic floor muscles. Your testicles will also rise when you contract these muscles.

Now that you know where these muscles are, contract them for 5 to 20 seconds. Then release them.

Repeat this exercise 10 to 20 times in a row, three to four times a day.

Exercise for Anus Muscles

Contracting and releasing of anus muscles daily 30 times a day in the morning, evening and night will strengthen the urinary bladder, pelvic and vaginal muscles and organs. Feel that air is entering via anus. Cosmic touch for organs

-**Men:** Do cosmic therapy for penis, testicles, and urinary bladder by holding them for 10 minutes for three times a day

-**Women:** Do cosmic therapy for the Vagina and Uterus by touching them for 10 minutes for three times a day.

This has worked for many people when medicines failed to arrest urination.

30.Erectile Dysfunction

Erectile dysfunction (ED) is the inability to get or keep an erection firm enough to
have sexual intercourse. It's also sometimes referred to as impotence. Occasional ED isn't uncommon. Many men experience it during times of stress. Frequent ED can be a sign of health problems that need treatment. It can also be a sign of emotional or relationship difficulties that may need to be addressed by a professional.
ED is not the only male sexual problem. Other types of male sexual dysfunction include:
Premature ejaculation
Delayed or absent ejaculation
Lack of interest in sex

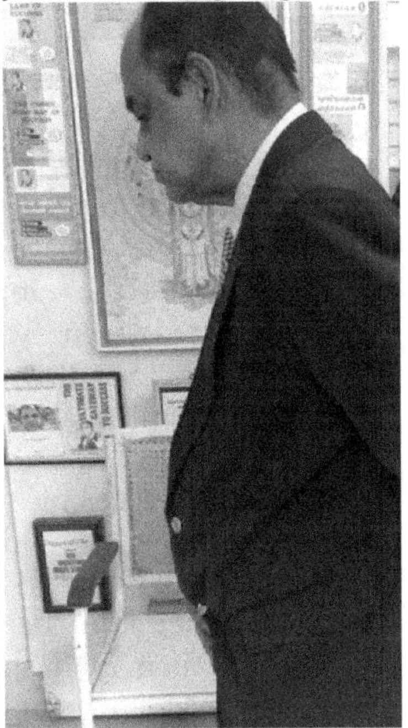

An erection is the result of increased blood flow into your penis. Blood flow is usually stimulated by either sexual thoughts or direct contact with your penis.

Kegel exercises are a simple exercise to stop frequent urination. This will strengthen your pelvic floor muscles. To do this, stop peeing midstream. The muscles you use to do this are your pelvic floor muscles. Your testicles will also rise when you contract these muscles.

Now that you know where these muscles are, contract them for 5 to 20 seconds. Then release them.
Repeat this exercise 10 to 20 times in a row, three to four times a day.

Exercise for Anus Muscles
Contracting and releasing of anus muscles daily 30 times a day in the morning, evening and night will strengthen the urinary bladder, pelvic and vaginal muscles and organs. Feel that air is entering via anus.
Cosmic touch for organs

-Men: Do cosmic therapy for penis, testicles, and urinary bladder by holding them for 10 minutes for three times a day
-Women: Do cosmic therapy for Vagina, Uterus by touching them for 10 minutes for three times a day.
This has worked for many people when medicines failed to arrest urination.

31.Premature Ejaculation

Premature ejaculation is a form of sexual dysfunction that can adversely affect the quality of a man's sex life. It is when an orgasm occurs sooner than wanted. In most cases, there is a psychological cause, and the prognosis is good.

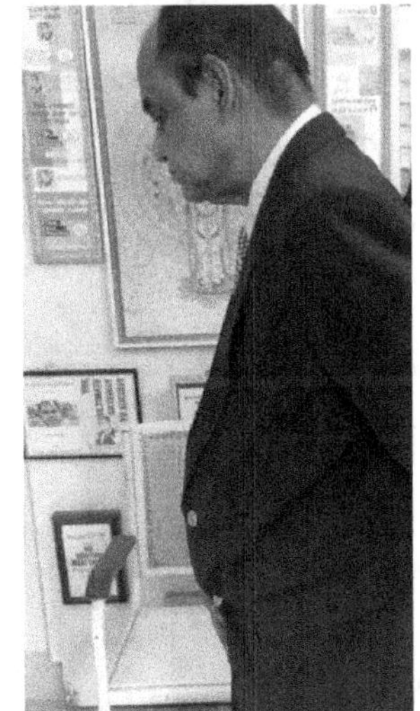

Kegel exercises are a simple exercise to stop frequent urination. This will strengthen your pelvic floor muscles. To do this, stop urinating midstream.

The muscles you use to do this are your pelvic floor muscles. Your testicles will also rise when you contract these muscles.

Now that you know where these muscles are, contract them for 5 to 20 seconds. Then release them.

Repeat this exercise 10 to 20 times in a row, three to four times a day.

Exercise for Anus Muscles and   organs

Contracting and releasing of anus muscles daily 30 times a day in the morning, evening and night will strengthen the urinary bladder, pelvic and vaginal muscles and organs. Feel that air is entering via anus.

Cosmic touch for organs

-Men: Do cosmic therapy for penis, testicles, and urinary bladder by holding them for 10 minutes for three times a day

-Women: Do cosmic therapy for Vagina, Uterus by touching them for 10 minutes for three times a day.

This has worked for many people when medicines failed to arrest urination.

4.My Formula for Success

My Formula to succeed: Energy + Thoughts = Achievement.

Energy is channelised through the hands. Thoughts refer to thinking and visualising. When these two forces join hands, they take you to success.

Everything should come from the depths of your heart and hence your actions should be oriented towards the target you strive for. Cosmic energy gives life for your dreams to materialise.

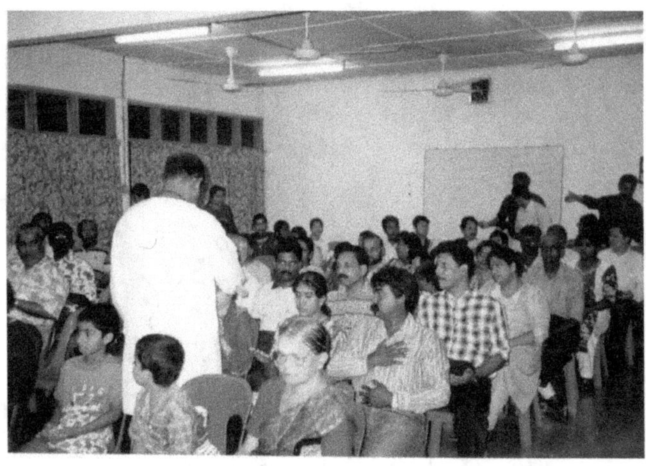

Avoid finding fault with others and refrain from the useless thought of analysing the reasons for failure. Energy flow is smooth when you start thinking that you alone are responsible for what you are now. Nature has only one aspect to offer, Abundance, and there is no secondary aspect called shortage. Adoption of cosmic energy is not confined to a particular time or day. It becomes imperative to conceive that this cosmic energy has already been attained voluntarily.

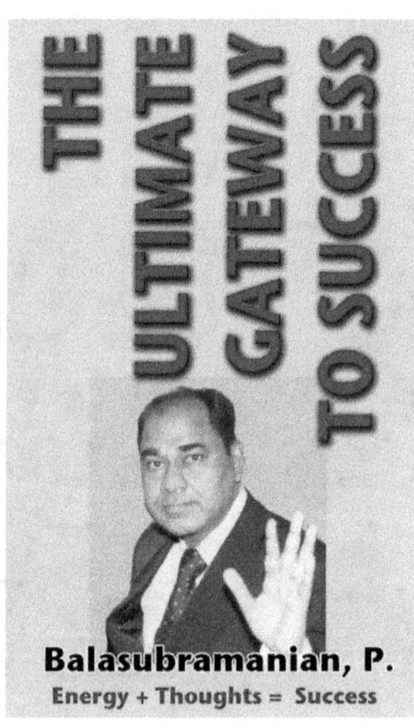

5. Ultimate Gateway to Success

Practice Bears Positive Results

My Desire

"This whole world should shine brighter. As light replaces darkness, we all should become lighted lamps."

A popular song now comes to my mind "Everyone has a good time and a bad patch in his life, and everyone is destined to be elevated and emancipated."

As a fitting conclusion, I quote a great poet saying, "I am not an incarnation to impart knowledge. Let us join hands as humans to create history."

Finally, "Energy plus Thought equals success" is the ultimate route to success.

* * *

6.Books by P.Balasubramanian

Technical Books
1. Energy Auditing Made Simple
2. How to make money through Energy Auditing –Vol.1 & 2
3. ISO Auditing Made Simple
4. Water scarcity and flood control

Personality Development books
1. The Ultimate Gateway of Success
2. Olimayamana Ethirkalam-Tamil (Part 1 & 2)
3. Reiki Sikichayin Ragasyangal – Tamil
4. Vanaveethiyil Oru Vetri Payanam – Tamil
5. Reiki Secrets Revealed
6. Future with Nature
7. Light the Lamp of success
8. Cosmic Road map of success
9. Energy Neuro Programming for Personality Development
10. Success in digital world